Contents

Introduction 4

Chapter one 5

What Is Coronary Heart Disease? 5

CHD vs. CAD vs. Atherosclerosis 6

Symptoms 7

Causes 9

What are risk factors for developing coronary heart disease? 9

Conventional Treatment 10

Natural Remedies for Coronary Heart Disease 11

7 days of heart healthy meals 23

Monday 23

Tuesday 23

Wednesday 24

Thursday 24

Friday 25

Saturday 25

Sunday 26

Chapter two 26

Anti-heart disease diet recipes 26

Winter Lentil Vegetable Soup 26

Instant Pot Lentil Vegetable Soup 29

Spicy Lentil Vegetable Soup 31

Chunky Vegetarian Vegetable Soup (Fast and Easy)..... 34

Chunky Tomato Potato Soup 36

Chunky Cheese Soup.. 37

Healthier Slow Cooker Chicken Stroganoff.................. 39

Low-Fat Sour Cream Chicken Enchiladas 41

Cottage Cheese Spinach Chicken 43

Cottage Meatloaf 45

Cottage Cheese Meatball Marinara 47

Vegetarian Cottage Cheese Patties.............................. 50

Strawberry and Spinach Salad with Honey Balsamic
Vinaigrette 52

Quinoa Vegetable Salad.. 54

Quinoa Salad with Dried Fruit and Nuts 56

Cucumber and Tomato Salad.. 58

Cherry Tomato Salad... 59

Tofu Sandwich Spread... 61

Baked Tofu Spinach Wrap... 63

Vegan Black Bean and Sweet Potato Salad................... 64

The Best Fresh Tomato Salsa 66

Easy Never Forgotten Guacamole 67

Amazing Chickpea Cinnamon Pancakes........................ 69

Crispy Jacket Potatoes 71

Conclusion.. 72

Introduction

Coronary heart disease (CHD) is currently the leading cause of death among adults in the U.S. — and according to the Centers For Disease Control and Prevention (CDC), it has maintained this ranking as the No. 1 killer since 1921.

Coronary heart disease is a condition caused by the buildup of waxy plaque in the arteries that flow to and from the heart. CHD often goes by several other names, including coronary artery disease, heart disease and arteriosclerotic heart disease.

What causes heart diseases, and what does this tell us about how to prevent it? Most cardiovascular disorders are related to elevated inflammation levels — so, as you'll learn, by reducing inflammation, the root of most diseases, you can place your body in a state that is conducive to healing.

Here's the good news for those struggling with heart disease: adjusting your diet, reducing stress levels and regularly exercising are all ways you can naturally control inflammation, and therefore are beneficial for treating and preventing coronary heart disease. And as you'll more about below, there are many whole foods that are available in common grocery stores that can help protect your heart, as well as lower your risk for developing various forms of chronic diseases in the future.

Chapter one

What Is Coronary Heart Disease?

CHD occurs when the small blood vessels that supply blood and oxygen to the heart narrow and sometimes harden, which over time can cause ruptures, heart attacks and other fatal conditions.

Heart disease is sometimes called a "disease of Western, modern civilization" because it was rare before 1900, and still remains much less common in pre-industrialized populations today. By the mid 1900s, coronary heart disease became the nation's biggest killer, and today all forms of cardiovascular diseases — including conditions of the heart and blood vessels like angina, congestive heart failure and stroke — are still the leading causes of death in many Western nations. Cardiovascular diseases kill more than 630,000 Americans a year, men and women pretty much equally. Currently, heart disease is the cause of about 1 in every 4 deaths in the U.S.

For the past several decades, doctors have mostly turned to medications and surgeries to help treat cardiovascular disease — including clot-busting prescription drugs, tiny balloons implanted inside the body to open up arteries and bypass surgeries.

The result is that, today, coronary heart disease is considered more chronic than necessarily fatal. However, these treatments are really resolving symptoms rather than addressing the underlying causes of heart disease. Recently, it's become apparent that lifestyle and dietary changes are fundamental to truly treating heart disease and/or preventing it from returning.

CHD vs. CAD vs. Atherosclerosis

Many people use the names coronary artery disease and coronary heart disease interchangeably.

Coronary artery disease is considered the most common type of heart disease. It occurs when there's a blockage of one or more arteries that supply blood to the heart.

In the first stage of heart disease, called angina, blood flow to the heart is restricted. When blood flow stops, there's a myocardial infarction, also known as a heart attack. The combination of these two conditions is what many doctors are referring to when they say "coronary heart disease" (or CHD).

What is atherosclerosis, and how does it differ from CHD/CAD? When someone has CHD or CAD, the buildup of substances inside their arteries is what is referred to as arteriosclerosis (also spelled atherosclerosis). The definition of arteriosclerosis is "a disease of the arteries characterized by the deposition of plaques of fatty material on their inner walls."

Arteriosclerosis refers to hardening and thickening of the walls of the arteries. It is often said to be "partly a function of aging." Over time the smooth, elastic arterial cells become more fibrous and stiff. Calcium, cholesterol particles and fatty acids accumulate on arterial walls and form a swelling called an atheroma. Atheroma are capable of bursting, causing blood clots, and leading to heart attacks or strokes. In populations that eat an unprocessed diet, far less inflammation-caused arteriosclerosis and heart disease are present.

Symptoms

Not everyone who has CHD even knows it — especially people who are in the early stages. Some symptoms of CHD can be very noticeable, however, it's also possible to have this disease and experience no symptoms at all or only slight symptoms.

Coronary artery disease symptoms vary a lot from person to person. The most common noticeable sign of CHD is having chest pain or discomfort, which is caused when the heart is not getting enough blood or oxygen.

Other coronary artery disease symptoms can include:

- Feeling a "heaviness" or like someone is squeezing your heart. This is called angina (another name for chest pain) and is probably the most common blocked artery symptom. It's possible to experience various forms of chest discomfort including heaviness, tightness, pressure, aching, burning, numbness or fullness.
- Pains or numbness in your breast bone (sternum), neck, arms, stomach or upper back
- Shortness of breath and fatigue with activity
- General weakness
- Indigestion or heartburn
- If CHD progresses, you may experience a heart attack, also called myocardial infarction. Heart attack symptoms can include:
- Pain or discomfort in the upper body including the chest, arms, left shoulder, back, neck, jaw or stomach
- Difficulty breathing and shortness of breath
- Sweating
- Feeling of fullness, indigestion, choking or heartburn

- Nausea or vomiting
- Light-headedness, dizziness and weakness
- Anxiety and panic
- Rapid or irregular heart beats

What really causes CHD and heart attacks? CHD is ultimately a result of inflammation from fatty material and other substances forming a buildup of plaque that accumulates within the walls of your arteries. Because these arteries have the crucial role of bringing blood and oxygen to your heart, reduced blood flow can slow down or stop your heartbeat, causing "cardiac arrest."

For this reason, medical professionals use a combination of lifestyle changes, medicines and medical procedures to slow, stop or reverse the buildup of plaque. This can help lower the risk of blood clots forming and a heart attack taking place because it widens clogged arteries.

What are risk factors for developing coronary heart disease?

- High amounts of free radical damage (also called oxidative stress) and low antioxidant levels in the body. When antioxidant levels are lower than those of free radicals due to poor nutrition and other lifestyle factors, oxidation wreaks havoc in the body — damaging cells, breaking down tissue, mutating DNA and overloading the immune system.

- Being a male, since men develop CHD more other than women (although it affects both sexes)
- Being over the age of 65
- High consumption of alcohol
- Smoking
- Eating a poor diet with unhealthy fats and processed foods
- Family history of coronary heart disease, stroke or peripheral arterial disease
- Menopause in women
- Having high blood pressure, diabetes or high cholesterol levels
- Lack of physical activity or exercise
- Obesity
- Sleep deprivation
- Exposure to environmental pollutants and toxic chemicals

Conventional Treatment

Half a century ago, coronary heart disease killed an even greater percentage of those who suffered from it, but fortunately, doctors today are more adept at using various treatments to control heart disease symptoms. Some of these are effective at lowering blood pressure, triglycerides and cholesterol, but many simply target symptoms and don't focus on the bigger picture.

Many doctors place people with coronary heart disease on a treatment plan that includes both prescription medications and lifestyle changes. Depending on which healthcare professional you choose, your symptoms and how severe the disease is, you might be prescribed one or more medicines to treat your high blood pressureor high cholesterol or to prevent complications like diabetes.

Examples of medications used to treat CHD include: cholesterol-modifying medications like aspirin, beta blockers, nitroglycerin, angiotensin-converting enzyme (ACE) inhibitors and angiotensin II receptor blockers (ARBs).

Many people are able to prevent CHD and recover from it naturally by maintaining a healthy lifestyle: changing their diet, stopping smoking, getting good sleep and adding in supplements on top of some other things we'll discuss below.

Natural Remedies for Coronary Heart Disease

Lifestyle Changes (Quitting Smoking & Eating A Healthy Diet)

A 2016 study found that living a healthy lifestyle — including exercising, eating a healthy diet full of fruits, vegetables and grains and not smoking — can lower your risk of heart disease, even if you are genetically predisposed to developing the disease. The study looked at 55,685 participants total in three prospective cohorts and one cross-sectional study. According to The New York Times:

The investigators found that genes can double the risk of heart disease, but a good lifestyle cuts it in half. Just as important, they found, a terrible lifestyle erases about half of the benefits of good genetics.

The individual results of each study were impressive. In the first study, when participants with the highest genetic risk followed a healthy lifestyle, they cut the 10-year likelihood of heart disease from 10.7 percent to 5.1 percent. In the second study, the high-risk and healthy lifestyle participants' 10-year risk dropped from 4.6 percent to 2 percent. In the third study, participants risk went from 8.2 percent to 5.3 percent. In the final study, participants with a high genetic risk living a healthy lifestyle had significantly less calcium in their coronary arteries, which is a sign of CHD.

This groundbreaking research illustrates that you can naturally reduce your risk of heart disease. Below we'll look closer at foods, supplements, essential oils and lifestyle changes you can implement to achieve greater health and fight off coronary heart disease.

Avoiding Inflammatory Foods

Should you eat a low-fat diet to prevent heart disease? When most people think of foods that increase their chances of developing heart disease, fatty cuts of meat and fried food probably come to mind. For many years, the public was led to believe that cholesterol-rich foods and saturated fats of all kinds increased the risk for heart disease. "The cholesterol hypothesis," as it's called, rested on the assumption that saturated fats raise cholesterol levels that wind up clogging the arteries.

However, a number of researchers today have demonstrated that this is not necessarily true, and that while this theory has been widely accepted, it has never been proven. Cholesterol is actually an essential component of healthy cells and organisms, and we all need to maintain a certain level to thrive!

According to a 2009 study published in the International Journal of Clinical Practice,

It is now acknowledged that the original studies purporting to show a linear relation between cholesterol intake and coronary heart disease (CHD)

may have contained fundamental study design flaws, including conflated cholesterol and saturated fat consumption rates and inaccurately assessed actual dietary intake of fats by study subjects.

Many experts today now believe that elevated blood cholesterol is a symptom, not a cause, of heart disease. Whether or not someone's blood cholesterol level is increased by eating a certain food depends on that person's individual cholesterol makeup, and each person is different. Several recent studies have shown that the dynamics of cholesterol homeostasis and of development of CHD are extremely complex and multifactorial. This suggests that the previously established relationship between dietary cholesterol and heart disease risk was overexaggerated.

In the majority of people, the real cause of heart disease may be inflammation. Foods to avoid to prevent CHD that promote inflammation include:

- Corn and soybean oils
- Pasteurized, conventional dairy
- Refined carbohydrates
- Conventional meat
- Sugars of all kinds
- Trans fats

But don't many health authorities still warn against eating too much fat? Despite the existing evidence that eating cholesterol isn't the cause of heart disease, most government-funded health associations, including the National Heart, Lung and Blood Institute, still recommend limiting saturated fats. As part of a treatment plan called "Therapeutic Lifestyle Changes" (TLC) — used to control high blood cholesterol through a healthy diet, physical activity and weight management — the Institute recommends that less than 7 percent of daily calories come from saturated fats. They recommend limiting fat-containing foods like meats, dairy products, chocolate, baked goods and deep-fried and processed foods.

The TLC diet is purposefully low in saturated fat, trans fat and dietary cholesterol. No more than 25–35 percent of your daily calories are intended to come from all fats, including saturated, trans, monounsaturated and polyunsaturated fats.

Going forward, we can expect guidelines like this to be updated to reflect the most recent study findings. Over the last decade, many countries and health promotion groups have modified their dietary recommendations to reflect the current evidence and, in fact, now address the negative consequence of ineffective dietary cholesterol in someone's diet.

Eating a Heart-Healthy Diet

Following a healthy, whole-foods–based diet can reduce inflammation, high blood pressure and unhealthy high cholesterol. Of course, eating well will also help you maintain a healthy weight and have more energy to be active, both of which are important for preventing coronary heart disease. Instead of focusing on eating low-fat foods to reduce fat and cholesterol, I believe we would be much better off making our goal to reduce inflammation.

The healthiest anti-inflammatory foods for fighting coronary heart disease are those brimming with antioxidants and phytonutrients that lower your immune system's overactive response. These help fight free radical damage and target the problem where it starts by lowering oxidative stress.

How do you know what the top antioxidant foods are? Anything loaded with fiber, grown directly from the earth and brightly colored is a good place to start!

Healthy fats and animal proteins have a place among other whole foods in a heart-healthy diet, too. When it comes to including healthy fats, the general effect of quality saturated fats in someone's diet is to help balance the ratio of HDL to LDL cholesterols. Regarding HDL cholesterol, some feel "the higher, the better," but we know that the ratio of cholesterol is important too.

Foods that help reduce inflammation and, therefore, the risk of CHD include:

Fiber-rich and antioxidant-rich foods of all kinds

Vegetables (all kinds, including beets, carrots, cruciferous vegetables like Brussels sprouts, broccoli, cabbage, cauliflower and kale, dark leafy greens, artichokes, onions, peas, salad greens, mushrooms, sea vegetables and squashes)

Fruits (all kinds, especially berries and citrus)

Herbs and spices, especially turmeric (curcumin) and raw garlic (also basil, chili peppers, cinnamon, curry powder, ginger, rosemary and thyme)

Traditional teas like green tea, oolong or white tea

Legumes and beans

Healthy fats found in nuts, seeds, avocados, wild-caught fish and extra virgin olive oil —learn about what high-cholesterol foods to avoid versus eat

Raw, unpasteurized dairy products, cage-free eggs and pasture-raised poultry

Red wine in moderation

If you look at evidence from many people living a traditional diet, it doesn't seem that saturated fats are the cause of coronary heart disease. Foods containing saturated fats — such as full-fat dairy, organ meats, beef, eggs, lard and butter — are actually found in high levels in many of the healthiest, longest-living people that have been studied, like those in the Blue Zones.

The Mediterranean diet is one of the most popular and effective anti-inflammatory diets that exists. Foods commonly eaten in the Mediterranean region include fish, vegetables, beans, fruits and olive oil. These have been shown to lower cholesterol and triglycerides and reduce symptoms of numerous chronic diseases. Following this type of diet that is low in sugar, processed foods, preservatives, vegetable oils and artificial ingredients can also help you maintain a healthier weight.

Using Heart-Healthy Supplements

You'll get the most benefits from a healthy diet when you consume real foods that provide natural, absorbable nutrients. While it's helpful to be aware of certain nutrients that can help protect your heart, eating a wide variety of whole foods and reducing toxin load in your body is by far the most important thing. That being said, some supplements added to a nutrient-dense diet may also be helpful for treating heart problems.

I recommend the following supplements for controlling inflammation and supporting heart health:

- Omega-3 fish oil supplements or 1 tablespoon of fish oil (such as cod liver oil) daily — if you avoid fish, try plant-based algal oil
- Curcumin (turmeric) and garlic supplements
- Coenzyme Q10
- Carotenoids
- Selenium
- Vitamin C
- Vitamin D
- Vitamin E
- Glucosamine

A study published in May, 2019 in the BMJ found evidence that habitual use of glucosamine supplements, which are commonly taken to help relieve osteoarthritis pain, may also be related to lower risks of cardiovascular disease (CVD) events. Ongoing use of glucosamine — which is a crystalline compound which is found inside connective tissue and cartilage — was associated with a 15 percent lower risk of total CVD events and a 9 to 22 percent lower risk of individual cardiovascular events. The protective effects of glucosamine on CVD outcomes were even stronger among current smokers.

The study followed over 466,000 participants without heart disease at the beginning of the study and tracked their supplement use and health for eight years. It was found that after adjusting for age, sex, body mass index, race, lifestyle factors, dietary intakes, drug use, and other supplement use, glucosamine use was associated with a significantly lower risk of total CVD events, CVD death, coronary heart disease development and stroke. It's believed glucosamine can reduce C reactive protein concentrations, which means it can help lower systemic inflammation, and also mimic the protective effects of a low-carbohydrate diet, since it can decrease glycolysis (the breakdown of glucose by enzymes) and increase breakdown of proteins.

Exercise

While there are really too many types and benefits of exercise to list here, just know that exercise helps restore and maintain cardiovascular health by improving blood flow, bringing more oxygen to your cells, managing hormones and blood sugar levels and helping you relax. This makes it one of the most powerful things you can to do prevent clogged arteries.

Studies suggest that exercise can benefit your heart just as much as certain medications. A meta-review of more than 305 clinical trials focusing on exercise benefits even found that, amazingly, no statistically detectable differences existed between those who exercised and those who were given medications in the prevention of coronary heart disease! The conclusion of the analysis was that "exercise and many drug interventions are often potentially similar in terms of their mortality benefits in the secondary prevention of coronary heart disease, rehabilitation after stroke, treatment of heart failure, and prevention of diabetes."

Try whichever type works best for you and your current level of fitness, such as burst training, HIIT workouts, Crossfit, yoga, Tai Chi or simply walking more.

Stress Reduction

Stress raises cortisol levels and may interfere with inflammatory responses when left unmanaged. Chronic stress caused by our modern, fast-paced lifestyles can affect just about every bodily system — suppressing the immune system, slowing metabolism, and stalling digestion, detoxification and cell regeneration.

Research conducted by the Department of Epidemiology and Public Health at University College of London suggests that:

Chronic stress predicts the occurrence of coronary heart disease (CHD). Employees who experience work-related stress and individuals who are socially isolated or lonely have an increased risk of a first CHD event … Among patients with CHD, acute psychological stress has been shown to induce transient myocardial ischemia and long-term stress can increase the risk of recurrent CHD events and mortality.

Some of the best natural stress relievers include nixing caffeine, smoking and alcohol, getting proper sleep, working out, praying and/or meditating, journaling, doing something creative, cooking or spending time with family and pets.

Essential Oils

There are many natural plant-derived essential oils that can help manage inflammation and symptoms related to heart disease. Some include lemongrass oil, helichrysum oil and ginger oil.

The active ingredients found in plants are their most potent in this concentrated form. Ginger essential oil, for example, contains the highest levels of anti-inflammatory gingerol, and helichrysum oil kicks off inflammatory enzyme inhibition, free-radical scavenging activity and corticoid-like effects. I recommend diffusing these oils in your home, inhaling them directly and applying them topically to your skin (such as over your chest) after mixing them with a carrier oil like coconut oil.

7 days of heart healthy meals

Monday

Lentil soup

Breakfast: Porridge made with skimmed milk and one sliced banana on top.

Lunch: Lentil and vegetable soup (spreads based on vegetable, olive or sunflower oil will be unsaturated so a better choice for your heart than butter).

Evening meal: One medium-sized jacket potato (cooked in the microwave or oven) with a tin of sardines in tomato sauce, served with peas.

Snacks: Two satsumas (or easy-peelers); one apple; a small handful of unsalted peanuts (30g); a serving (125g) of fat-free Greek-style yoghurt.

Tuesday

Chunky vegetable goulash

Breakfast: Two slices of wholegrain toast with spread, one boiled egg and a sliced medium tomato.

Lunch: Carrot and parsnip soup (use leftovers if you made Monday's recipe, or make fresh with extra portions to freeze); two slices of wholemeal bread with spread.

Evening meal: Homemade chunky vegetable and bean goulash (pictured); brown rice; broccoli.

Snacks: Three oatcakes with low-fat cream cheese or quark; one pear.

Wednesday

Breakfast: No-added-sugar muesli with skimmed milk, topped with one sliced banana.

Lunch: Jacket potato with half a can of reduced-sugar-and-salt baked beans; a portion of salad.

Evening meal: Beetroot barley risotto (pictured); served with peas.

Snacks: One carrot cut into sticks; a small handful of unsalted peanuts; two satsumas.

Thursday

Breakfast: Two slices of wholegrain toast with spread, sliced or mashed banana, and a serving of fat-free Greek-style yoghurt.

Lunch: Egg, tomato and cucumber wholemeal bread sandwich.

Evening meal: Wholewheat spaghetti with sardines and cherry tomatoes; a portion of salad.

Snacks: Two plums; two oatcakes with spread; one pear.

Friday

Mushroom and cauliflower frittata

Breakfast: No-added-sugar muesli with skimmed milk and a banana.

Lunch: Cheese salad sandwich made with reduced-fat Cheddar, salad, two slices of wholegrain bread and spread.

Evening meal: Homemade mushroom and cauliflower frittata, served with peas and carrots or any other leftover/surplus vegetables.

Snacks: Two plums; two oatcakes with spread; one pear.

Saturday

Tuna and sweetcorn pasta bake

Breakfast: Porridge made with skimmed milk; one banana.

Lunch: Vegetable soup

Evening meal: Homemade tuna and sweetcorn pasta bake, served with cauliflower and broccoli.

Snacks: Small handful of unsalted peanuts, one apple, one pear..

Sunday

Chicken and vegetable traybake

Breakfast: Poached egg and a portion of cooked mushrooms, with two slices of wholemeal bread.

Lunch: Chicken and vegetable traybake (pictured); baked apple with spiced sultanas and low-fat custard or homemade custard with low-fat milk.

Evening meal: Chicken, cucumber and tomato wholemeal bread sandwiches (using leftovers from the lunchtime traybake).

Snacks: Small handful of unsalted peanuts; one carrot cut into sticks; two satsumas (or easy-peelers).

Chapter two

Anti-heart disease diet recipes

Winter Lentil Vegetable Soup

This soup has very little fat, is cheap and easy to make and delicious. Our family practically lives on it in the winter and I usually double the recipe. Sprinkle grated cheddar on top if you wish. If you can't hang around long enough for this to cook, put it in a slow cooker.

Prep Time: 20 mins

Cook Time: 1 hr 30 mins

Additional Time: 1 hr 10 mins

Total Time: 3 hrs

Servings: 6

Yield: 6 to 1 - cup servings

Ingredients

½ cup red or green lentils

1 cup chopped onion

1 stalk celery, chopped

2 cups shredded cabbage

1 (28 ounce) can whole peeled tomatoes, chopped

2 cups chicken broth

3 carrots, chopped

1 clove garlic, crushed

1 teaspoon salt

½ teaspoon ground black pepper

¼ teaspoon white sugar

½ teaspoon dried basil

½ teaspoon dried thyme

¼ teaspoon curry powder

Directions

Place the lentils into a stockpot or a Dutch oven and add water to twice the depth of the lentils. Bring to a boil, then lower heat and let simmer for about 15 minutes. Drain and rinse lentils; return them to the pot.

Add onion, celery, cabbage, tomatoes, chicken broth, carrots and garlic to the pot and season with salt, pepper, sugar, basil, thyme and curry. Cook, simmering for 1 1/2 to 2 hours or until desired tenderness is achieved.

Cook's Note:

Combine ingredients in a slow cooker and cook on Low for 8 to 10 hours, or on High for about 4 hours, or until lentils have broken down and vegetables are tender.

Easy Cleanup

Try using a liner in your slow cooker for easier cleanup.

Nutrition Facts (per serving)

112 Calories, 1g Fat, 22g Carbs, 6g Protein

Instant Pot Lentil Vegetable Soup

Warm and healthy one-pot dish cooked in an Instant Pot.

Prep Time: 20 mins

Cook Time: 40 mins

Additional Time: 5 min

Total Time: 1 hr 5 mins

Servings: 8

Ingredients

1 teaspoon vegetable oil

1 large onion, chopped

1 red bell pepper, chopped

1 carrot, chopped

3 cloves garlic, minced

4 (14.5 ounce) cans chicken broth

1 pound lentils, rinsed and drained

2 medium zucchini, chopped

1 small eggplant, peeled and chopped

1 (14 ounce) can diced tomatoes with juice

1 tablespoon dried parsley

2 teaspoons ground cumin

1 teaspoon salt

2 teaspoons lemon zest

1 tablespoon lemon juice

Directions

Place oil in a multi-functional pressure cooker (such as Instant Pot) and select Saute function. Add onion, bell pepper, and carrot; cook and stir until the onion has softened and turned translucent, about 5 minutes. Stir in garlic and saute until fragrant, about 1 minute. Cancel Saute function.

Add chicken broth, lentils, zucchini, eggplant, diced tomatoes with juice, parsley, cumin, and salt to the pot. Close and lock the lid. Select high pressure according to manufacturer's instructions; set timer for 20 minutes. Allow 10 to 15 minutes for pressure to build.

Release pressure carefully using the quick-release method according to manufacturer's instructions, about 5 minutes. Unlock and remove the lid. Stir in lemon juice and zest.

Tips

To make this vegetarian, use vegetable broth in place of chicken broth.

Spicy Lentil Vegetable Soup

This is a healthy, hearty, spicy, relatively easy-to-make, delicious soup recipe. The roasted peppers really make it something special. I just made it up and am eating it now, and I am in love.

Prep Time: 20 mins

Cook Time: 50 mins

Additional Time 20 mins

Total Time: 1 hr 30 mins

Servings: 4

Yield: 4 servings

Ingredients

1 red bell pepper

½ green bell pepper

3 cups water

1 cup brown lentils

1 tablespoon olive oil

1 carrot, sliced

1 onion, chopped

1 broccoli floret, chopped

2 cups vegetable broth

1 tablespoon crushed red pepper flakes

1 tablespoon ground ginger

1 tablespoon ground black pepper

1 teaspoon dried thyme leaves

1 teaspoon dried rubbed sage

Directions

Preheat an oven to 375 degrees F (190 degrees C). Line a baking sheet with aluminum foil.

Cut the peppers in half from top to bottom; remove the stem, seeds, and ribs, then place the peppers cut-side-down onto the prepared baking sheet.

Bake in the preheated oven until limp, 30 to 40 minutes. Turn the peppers over halfway through cooking. Once ready, place the peppers into a bowl, and tightly seal with plastic wrap. Allow the peppers to steam as they cool, about 20 minutes. Once cool, remove the skins and discard. Chop the peppers

Meanwhile, bring the water and lentils to a boil in a saucepan over high heat. Reduce heat to medium-low, cover, and simmer until the lentils are tender, about 30 minutes. Drain, rinse, and set aside.

Heat the olive oil in a large saucepan over medium heat. Stir in the carrot, onion, and broccoli; cook and stir until the onion has softened, about 5 minutes. Pour in some of the vegetable broth, cover, and steam the vegetables until tender. Pour in the remaining vegetable broth and chopped peppers; season with the red pepper flakes, ginger, black pepper, thyme, and sage. Simmer until the flavors come together and the vegetables are very tender, about 20 to 30 minutes. Add water if needed to maintain your desired consistency. Stir in the cooked lentils until hot.

If desired, pour the soup into a blender, filling the pitcher no more than halfway full. Hold down the lid of the blender with a folded kitchen towel, and carefully start the blender, using a few quick pulses to get the soup moving before leaving it on to puree. Puree in batches until smooth and pour into a clean pot. Alternately, you can use a stick blender and puree the soup right in the cooking pot.

Cook's Note

To cut the time of this recipe in half, don't roast the peppers, add them to the saucepan when frying the other vegetables. Use ready-to-eat, canned lentils.

Chunky Vegetarian Vegetable Soup (Fast and Easy)

I make this super-easy vegetarian vegetable soup about every other week. It's thick and hearty, almost like a stew. Served with warm whole grain bread it makes a filling meal. Use green peas or green peas in place of okra if preferred.

Prep Time: 15 mins

Cook Time: 35 mins

Total Time: 50 mins

Servings: 10

Yield: 10 servings

Ingredients

2 tablespoons olive oil

½ onion, chopped

3 stalks celery, chopped

2 cloves garlic, minced

4 cups vegetable broth

1 (15 ounce) can tomato sauce

4 carrots, peeled and cut into 1/4-inch rounds

2 baking potatoes, cut into bite-size pieces

1 cup frozen corn

1 cup frozen shelled edamame (green soybeans)

1 cup frozen sliced okra

2 leaves kale, roughly chopped

salt to taste

1 teaspoon ground black pepper

Directions

Heat olive oil in a large pot over medium heat. Cook and stir onion and celery in hot oil until onion is softened and translucent, about 5 minutes.

Stir garlic into the onion mixture; cook and stir until fragrant, 2 to 3 minutes more.

Pour vegetable broth and tomato sauce into pot. Simmer for about 10 minutes.

Stir carrots and potatoes through the broth. Simmer until carrots are tender, 10 to 15 minutes more.

Drop corn, edamame, okra, and kale into the soup. Continue to simmer until okra is tender, 5 to 10 minutes more. Season with salt and pepper.

Cook's Note

For the vegetable broth, I use two no-salt-added vegan bouillon cubes and four cups of water. I don't add any salt to the soup while it's cooking so everyone can salt their own bowl.

Chunky Tomato Potato Soup

Creamy soup filled with chunky vegetables.

Prep Time: 20 mins

Cook Time: 35 mins

Total Time: 55 mins

Servings: 8

Yield: 8 servings

Ingredients

2 tablespoons butter

2 onions, chopped

4 cups peeled, cubed potatoes

1 ½ cups chopped celery

1 ½ cups chopped carrots

2 cloves garlic, minced

1 tablespoon Italian seasoning

2 cups milk

1 tablespoon cornstarch

1 (14.5 ounce) can tomatoes

1 ¼ cups chicken broth

2 tablespoons tomato paste

salt and pepper to taste

Directions

Melt the butter in a large saucepan over medium heat, and cook the onions until tender. Mix in the potatoes, celery, carrots, and garlic. Season with Italian seasoning. Pour in milk, gradually stir in cornstarch, and bring to a boil. Mix in tomatoes, broth, and tomato paste. Return to boil, reduce heat to low, and simmer 20 minutes. Season with salt and pepper.

Chunky Cheese Soup

A Cheddar cheese soup filled with chunks of vegetables and ham.

Prep Time: 20 mins

Cook Time: 40 mins

Total Time: 1 hr

Servings: 8

Yield: 8 servings

Ingredients

2 cups water

2 cups peeled and diced potatoes

½ cup diced carrots

½ cup chopped celery

¼ cup chopped onions

1 ½ teaspoons salt

¼ teaspoon ground black pepper

1 cup cooked ham, cubed

¼ cup butter

¼ cup all-purpose flour

2 cups milk

2 cups shredded Cheddar cheese

Directions

In a large saucepan, mix the water, potatoes, carrots, celery, onions, salt and pepper. Bring to boil. Reduce heat and simmer 30 minutes, or until vegetables are tender.

Mix the ham into the vegetable mixture.

In a medium saucepan, melt the butter. Stir in the flour until smooth. Slowly pour in the milk. Bring to a boil. Cook and stir 2 minutes, or until thickened. Stir in the Cheddar cheese until melted.

Mix the melted cheese mixture with the vegetable mixture and serve.

Healthier Slow Cooker Chicken Stroganoff

Cubed chicken breast cooked in the slow cooker with a creamy sauce mixture. This healthier version includes peas, low-fat cream cheese, butter instead of margarine, and natural cream of chicken soup. You also make your own seasoning mix instead of using a packaged mix. Serve over hot cooked rice or noodles, if desired.

Prep Time: 10 mins

Cook Time: 5 hrs 30 mins

Total Time: 5 hrs 40 mins

Servings: 4

Yield: 4 servings

Ingredients

1 tablespoon chopped carrot

1 tablespoon chopped parsley

1 tablespoon chopped onion

1 clove garlic

¼ teaspoon lemon zest

1 teaspoon salt

¼ teaspoon ground black pepper

4 skinless, boneless chicken breast halves - cubed

2 tablespoons butter

4 ounces Neufchatel cheese

8 ounces natural cream of chicken soup

1 cup frozen peas

Directions

Combine the carrot, parsley, onion, garlic, lemon zest, salt, and ground pepper in a small blender or food processor. Process until finely chopped and transfer to slow cooker. Add chicken and butter and mix. Cook on Low for 5 to 6 hours.

Stir in Neufchatel cheese, chicken soup, and peas. Cook on High until heated through, about 30 minutes.

Editor's Note:

This recipe is a healthier version of Slow Cooker Chicken Stroganoff.

Low-Fat Sour Cream Chicken Enchiladas

I had been looking for a recipe for restaurant-quality enchiladas with sour cream sauce, and my friend's grandma gave me this one that's made with ingredients that are lower in fat and calories. It's so simple to make! If you don't like really spicy foods, the optional items listed can be removed from the recipe and the dish is just as yummy.

Prep Time: 20 mins

Cook Time: 35 mins

Total Time: 55 mins

Servings: 8

Yield: 8 enchiladas

Ingredients

1 (16 ounce) container fat-free sour cream

1 (10.5 ounce) can condensed reduced-fat cream of chicken soup

1 tablespoon chopped fresh cilantro (Optional)

cooking spray (such as Pam®)

1 (10 ounce) can diced tomatoes with green chile peppers (such as RO*TEL®)

1 cup shredded cooked chicken, or more to taste

1 cup chopped onion (Optional)

1 (4 ounce) can diced green chiles (Optional)

8 (8 inch) flour tortillas, warmed

2 cups shredded Colby-pepperjack cheese, divided

Directions

Mix sour cream, condensed soup, and cilantro in a saucepan over medium heat; cook, stirring occasionally, until heated through, 3 to 5 minutes. Remove from the heat.

Spray a large skillet with cooking spray; add diced tomatoes, chicken, onion, and green chiles. Cook and stir over medium heat until onion is transparent, 5 to 10 minutes.

Preheat the oven to 350 degrees F (175 degrees C). Spray an 8x11-inch baking dish with cooking spray.

Spoon 2 to 3 tablespoons chicken mixture down the center of each warm tortilla, then sprinkle with about

1 tablespoon pepper Jack cheese. Roll each tortilla around filling and place seam-side down into the prepared baking dish. Pour sour cream sauce over tortillas and sprinkle remaining cheese over top.

Bake in the preheated oven until sauce is bubbling and cheese is melted, 25 to 30 minutes.

Cottage Cheese Spinach Chicken

Cajun-seasoned chicken breast stuffed with a cottage cheese and spinach mixture, then baked in butter. Serve with tossed salad, if desired.

Prep: 10 mins

Cook: 25 mins

Total: 35 mins

Servings: 4

Yield: 4 servings

Ingredients

1 (10 ounce) package frozen chopped spinach, thawed

½ yellow onion, chopped

1 cup cottage cheese

4 skinless, boneless chicken breast halves

2 tablespoons Cajun-style seasoning

2 tablespoons melted butter

Directions

Step 1

Preheat oven to 350 degrees F (175 degrees C).

Step 2

Squeeze excess water out of thawed spinach; in a large bowl, mix spinach with onion and cottage cheese and set aside.

Step 3

Season chicken breasts with Cajun-style seasoning, then place 1/4 of cheese/spinach mixture in the center of each breast and fold in half. Secure with toothpicks and place in a lightly greased 9x13 inch baking dish.

Step 4

Drizzle with melted butter and bake at 350 degrees F (175 degrees C) for about 25 minutes, or until chicken is cooked through and juices run clear.

Nutrition Facts

Per Serving: 274 calories; protein 37.4g; carbohydrates 7.5g; fat 10.4g; cholesterol 92.1mg; sodium 1109.5mg.

Garnish with fresh herbs, if desired.

Prep: 15 mins

Cook: 45 mins

Additional: 5 mins

Total: 1 hr 5 mins

Servings: 8

Yield: 1 - 9x5 inch loaf

Ingredients

Meatloaf:

1 ½ pounds lean ground beef

½ cup ketchup

⅓ cup tomato juice

½ teaspoon salt

½ teaspoon ground black pepper

⅛ teaspoon crushed red pepper

2 eggs, beaten

¾ cup fresh bread crumbs

¼ cup diced onion

2 teaspoons prepared mustard

Topping:

½ cup ketchup

1 teaspoon prepared mustard

4 teaspoons brown sugar

Directions

Step 1

Preheat oven to 400 degrees F (200 degrees C). Line a 9x5-inch loaf pan with aluminum foil.

Step 2

In a large bowl, combine ground beef, ketchup, tomato juice, salt, pepper, red pepper, eggs, bread crumbs, onion, and mustard for meatloaf until well mixed. Press meat mixture into the prepared pan.

Step 3

In a separate bowl, combine ketchup, mustard, and brown sugar for topping until smooth. Spread brown sugar mixture over meatloaf.

Step 4

Bake in preheated oven 35 to 45 minutes, until no longer pink. Drain off fat. Let rest 5 minutes before serving.

Nutrition Facts

Per Serving: 326 calories; protein 18.7g; carbohydrates 18.3g; fat 19.6g; cholesterol 110.3mg; sodium 679.9mg.

Cottage Cheese Meatball Marinara

The quest to make a healthier meatball has been a challenge. Often using leaner ground meats leads to tough and dry meatballs. Cottage cheese is the 'secret' ingredient that keeps these better-for-you meatballs moist and delicious. Share the fun and host a weekend meatball party. Invite your friends over to make big batches of these tasty, oven-baked meatballs to fill everyone's freezer with a quick weeknight meal solution.

Prep: 25 mins

Cook: 45 mins

Total: 1 hr 10 mins

Servings: 6

Yield: 6 servings

Ingredients

1 cup Nordica 2% Cottage Cheese

½ cup plain dry breadcrumbs

¼ cup grated Ivanhoe Parmesan Cheese, or as needed

3 cloves garlic, minced and divided

2 eggs, lightly beaten

½ teaspoon salt

½ teaspoon pepper

1 pound extra lean ground beef

1 mild Italian pork sausage, casing removed

3 cups passata or pureed, strained tomatoes

½ cup grated onion

Pinch hot pepper flakes

½ cup chopped fresh basil leaves

Directions

Step 1

Preheat the oven to 425 degrees F (220 degrees C). Stir the cottage cheese with the breadcrumbs, Parmesan cheese, 1 clove garlic, eggs and half each of the salt and pepper until well combined. Crumble in the ground beef and sausage meat; gently mix until well combined.

Step 2

Shape the mixture into 24 equal-sized meatballs; arrange, in a single layer, in a 9 x 13-inch (3 L) baking dish. Bake for 15 minutes or until lightly browned and set.

Step 3

Meanwhile, stir the passata with the grated onion, hot pepper flakes, remaining garlic, salt and pepper. Pour the tomato mixture evenly over the meatballs and cook for 30 minutes or until meatballs are cooked through and sauce is slightly thickened; gently stir in basil. Serve with additional Parmesan cheese to taste. Serve meatballs over hot cooked pasta or rice.

To shorten the prep time, make 12 large meatballs instead the small ones.

Spoon the meatballs into long buns and top with shredded mozzarella or provolone cheese for a meatball submarine sandwich.

Recipe doubles or triples easily to serve a crowd.

Increase hot pepper flakes to taste for a spicier sauce.

Make ahead: After baking the meatballs for 15 minutes, cool slightly and transfer to an air-tight container along with the uncooked sauce. Reserve in the refrigerator for 1 day or freeze for up to 3 months. Thaw in the refrigerator overnight. Cook for 30 to 40 minutes or until bubbly and thickened.

Nutrition Facts

Per Serving: 310 calories; protein 27g; carbohydrates 17.8g; fat 14.7g; cholesterol 121.6mg; sodium 1205.8mg.

Vegetarian Cottage Cheese Patties

Delicious addition to any menu. Don't be scared of the name. I hate cottage cheese but love these.

Prep: 10 mins

Cook: 25 mins

Total: 35 mins

Servings: 8

Yield: 8 servings

Ingredients

3 eggs

1 ½ cups cottage cheese

1 ½ cups quick rolled oats

3 tablespoons wheat germ (Optional)

1 (1 ounce) envelope dry onion soup mix

1 teaspoon dried thyme

2 tablespoons vegetable oil (for frying)

1 (10 ounce) can condensed cream of mushroom soup

Directions

Step 1

Preheat oven to 350 degrees F (175 degrees C).

Step 2

Beat eggs into a large bowl. Stir in cottage cheese, rolled oats, wheat germ, dry onion soup mix, and dried thyme. Form into 8 patties.

Step 3

Heat oil in a skillet over medium heat. Place patties in oil, and brown on both sides. Remove patties to a 9x13-inch baking dish.

Step 4

Pour condensed soup into a small bowl. Stir in 1/2 can of water (or milk) to dilute, then pour over patties.

Step 5

Bake in a preheated oven until the soup is bubbly, about 20 minutes.

Nutrition Facts

Per Serving: 180 calories; protein 11.1g; carbohydrates 17.6g; fat 7.5g; cholesterol 76.1mg; sodium 736.7mg.

Strawberry and Spinach Salad with Honey Balsamic Vinaigrette

This is a great easy summer salad, with a lot of options as to mixing and matching. Plus the salad looks pretty fancy. You can throw in any summer fruit or berry with this mix, blueberries and raspberries are a good choice, as are blackberries later in the season. The nuts are optional but a pecan or roasted almond adds a little crunch and more protein!

Prep: 15 mins

Total: 15 mins

Servings: 4

Yield: 4 servings

Ingredients

1 bunch fresh spinach

1 cup sliced fresh strawberries

½ cup crumbled Gorgonzola cheese

½ cup raw pecans

¼ cup balsamic vinegar

2 tablespoons honey

½ cup olive oil

salt and ground black pepper to taste

Directions

Step 1

Combine the spinach, strawberries, Gorgonzola cheese, and pecans in a large bowl.

Step 2

Stir the balsamic vinegar and honey together in a bowl; slowly stream the olive oil into the mixture while whisking continuously. Season with salt and pepper. Drizzle the dressing over the salad just before serving.

Nutrition Facts

Per Serving: 491 calories; protein 8.7g; carbohydrates 19.3g; fat 44.2g; cholesterol 22.5mg; sodium 282.4mg.

This is a wonderful dish--light and very tasty! My four kids (ages 2-7) ate it up and asked for more!

Prep: 20 mins

Cook: 25 mins

Additional: 45 mins

Total: 1 hr 30 mins

Servings: 12

Yield: 5 cups

Ingredients

1 teaspoon canola oil

1 tablespoon minced garlic

¼ cup diced (yellow or purple) onion

2 ½ cups water

2 teaspoons salt, or to taste

¼ teaspoon ground black pepper

2 cups quinoa

¾ cup diced fresh tomato

¾ cup diced carrots

½ cup diced yellow bell pepper

½ cup diced cucumber

½ cup frozen corn kernels, thawed

¼ cup diced red onion

1 ½ tablespoons chopped fresh cilantro

1 tablespoon chopped fresh mint

1 teaspoon salt

¼ teaspoon ground black pepper

2 tablespoons olive oil

3 tablespoons balsamic vinegar

Directions

Step 1

Heat the canola oil in a saucepan over medium heat. Cook and stir the garlic and 1/4 cup onion in the hot oil until the onion has softened and turned translucent, about 5 minutes. Pour in the water, 2 teaspoons salt, and 1/4 teaspoon black pepper and bring to a boil; stir the quinoa into the mixture, reduce heat to medium-low, and cover. Simmer until the quinoa is tender, about 20 minutes. Drain any remaining water from the quinoa with a mesh strainer and transfer to a large mixing bowl. Refrigerate until cold.

Step 2

Stir the tomato, carrots, bell pepper, cucumber, corn, and 1/4 cup red onion into the chilled quinoa. Season with cilantro, mint, 1 teaspoon salt, and 1/4 teaspoon black pepper. Drizzle the olive oil and balsamic vinegar over the salad; gently stir until evenly mixed.

Nutrition Facts

Per Serving: 148 calories; protein 4.6g; carbohydrates 22.9g; fat 4.5g; sodium 592.1mg.

Quinoa Salad with Dried Fruit and Nuts

This is an unusual and tasty high-protein grain salad. Quinoa is a grain that has almost no flavor, but the spices add zest. It's well worth trying, I make it often since discovering quinoa at my health food store.

Prep: 20 mins

Cook: 20 mins

Additional: 1 hr 20 mins

Total: 2 hrs

Servings: 10

Yield: 5 cups

Ingredients

1 ½ cups quinoa

¼ teaspoon salt

3 ½ cups water

1 bunch green onions, chopped

¾ cup chopped celery

½ cup raisins

1 pinch cayenne pepper

1 tablespoon vegetable oil

1 tablespoon distilled white vinegar

2 tablespoons lemon juice

2 tablespoons sesame oil

⅓ cup chopped fresh cilantro

¾ cup chopped pecans

Directions

Step 1

Bring the quinoa, salt, and water to a boil in a saucepan. Reduce heat to medium-low, cover, and simmer until the quinoa is tender, 20 to 25 minutes. Once done, scrape into a large bowl, and allow to cool for 20 minutes. Stir in the green onions, celery, raisins, cayenne pepper, vegetable oil, vinegar, lemon juice, and sesame oil. Allow to stand at room temperature for 1 hour to allow the flavors to blend. Stir in the cilantro and pecans before serving.

Nutrition Facts

Per Serving: 221 calories; protein 5.1g; carbohydrates 26.3g; fat 11.6g; sodium 71.9mg.

Cucumber and Tomato Salad

A refreshing, light salad for any hot, humid summer day! The kidney beans and tofu make it a great main dish for vegetarians, as well. The basil may be substituted with fresh parsley or mint. Be sure to make this salad just before serving.

Prep: 15 mins

Total: 15 mins

Servings: 4

Yield: 4 servings

Ingredients

1 tomato, chopped

1 cucumber, seeded and chopped

¼ cup thinly sliced red onion

¼ cup canned kidney beans, drained

¼ cup diced firm tofu

2 tablespoons chopped fresh basil

¼ cup balsamic vinaigrette salad dressing

salt and pepper to taste

Directions

Step 1

In a large bowl, combine the tomato, cucumber, red onion, kidney beans, tofu, and basil. Just before serving, toss with balsamic vinaigrette salad dressing, and season with salt and pepper.

Nutrition Facts

Per Serving: 98 calories; protein 4.1g; carbohydrates 8.6g; fat 6.1g; sodium 214.8mg.

Cherry Tomato Salad

This recipe was passed on by a friend and has been passed on to many more friends. It is a colorful and delicious salad served in a self-made vinaigrette. Always an excellent choice when entertaining for dinner.

Prep: 15 mins

Cook: 5 mins

Additional: 1 hr

Total: 1 hr 20 mins

Servings: 6

Yield: 6 servings

Ingredients

40 cherry tomatoes, halved

1 cup pitted and sliced green olives

1 (6 ounce) can black olives, drained and sliced

2 green onions, minced

3 ounces pine nuts

½ cup olive oil

2 tablespoons red wine vinegar

1 tablespoon white sugar

1 teaspoon dried oregano

Salt and pepper to taste

Directions

Step 1

In a big bowl, combine cherry tomatoes, green olives, back olives, and spring onion.

Step 2

In a dry skillet, toast pine nuts over medium heat until golden brown, turning frequently. Stir into tomato mixture.

Step 3

In a small bowl, mix together olive oil, red wine vinegar, sugar, and oregano. Season to taste with salt and pepper. Pour over salad, and gently stir to coat. Chill for 1 hour.

Nutrition Facts

Per Serving: 341 calories; protein 5.1g; carbohydrates 12.6g; fat 32.2g; sodium 939.9mg.

Tofu Sandwich Spread

This is a favorite vegetarian sandwich spread made with tofu. Makes a great sandwich filling or you can eat it with crackers.

Prep: 15 mins

Total: 15 mins

Servings: 4

Yield: 4 servings

Ingredients

1 pound firm tofu

1 stalk celery, chopped

1 green onion, chopped

½ cup mayonnaise

2 tablespoons soy sauce

1 tablespoon lemon juice

Directions

Step 1

Drain the block of tofu, and freeze overnight. Thaw, and cut into quarters. Squeeze out any moisture by hand, then wrap in paper towels, and squeeze again. Crumble into a medium bowl.

Step 2

Add celery and green onion to the tofu. Stir in mayonnaise, soy sauce and lemon juice until well blended.

Nutrition Facts

Per Serving: 370 calories; protein 18.8g; carbohydrates 7.2g; fat 31.8g; cholesterol 10.4mg; sodium 631.7mg.

These are quick, simple and tasty! My husband, who previously hated tofu (although this was deli style tofu), loved them and asked for more.

Prep: 3 mins

Cook: 2 mins

Total: 5 mins

Servings: 2

Yield: 2 wraps

Ingredients

2 (10 inch) whole wheat tortillas

1 (7.5 ounce) package hickory flavor baked tofu

½ cup shredded sharp Cheddar cheese

1 cup fresh baby spinach

1 tablespoon Ranch dressing

1 tablespoon grated Parmesan cheese, or to taste

Directions

Step 1

Place the tortillas side by side on a paper plate. Slice tofu, and place slices down the center of each tortilla.

Sprinkle cheese over the tofu. Cover with a damp paper towel, and heat in the microwave for about 45 seconds, or until cheese is melted.

Step 2

Pile some spinach onto each tortilla, and pour on some Ranch dressing. Sprinkle with Parmesan cheese, roll tortillas around the filling, and eat.

Nutrition Facts

Per Serving: 449 calories; protein 35.2g; carbohydrates 33.9g; fat 20.4g; cholesterol 40.4mg; sodium 567.2mg.

Vegan Black Bean and Sweet Potato Salad

This is a great side dish using fresh ingredients. There are never leftovers!

Prep: 15 mins

Cook: 25 mins

Total: 40 mins

Servings: 4

Yield: 4 servings

Ingredients

1 pound sweet potatoes, peeled and cut into 3/4-inch cubes

3 tablespoons olive oil, divided

½ teaspoon ground cumin, or more to taste

¼ teaspoon red pepper flakes (Optional)

coarse salt and ground black pepper to taste

2 tablespoons freshly squeezed lime juice

1 (14.5 ounce) can black beans, rinsed and drained

½ red onion, finely chopped

½ cup chopped fresh cilantro

Directions

Step 1

Preheat oven to 450 degrees F (230 degrees C).

Step 2

Spread sweet potatoes onto a rimmed baking sheet. Drizzle 1 tablespoon olive oil over sweet potatoes; season with cumin, red pepper flakes, salt, and pepper. Toss sweet potatoes until evenly coated.

Step 3

Roast on the lower rack of the preheated oven, stirring halfway through, until sweet potatoes are tender, 25 to 35 minutes.

Step 4

Whisk remaining 2 tablespoons olive oil and lime juice together in a large bowl; season with salt and pepper. Add sweet potatoes, black beans, onion, and cilantro; gently toss to coat.

Nutrition Facts

Per Serving: 291 calories; protein 8.4g; carbohydrates 42.2g; fat 10.6g; sod

The Best Fresh Tomato Salsa

Great with your favorite chips. Gets better as the flavors meld.

Prep: 20 mins

Total: 20 mins

Servings: 44

Yield: 5 cups

Ingredients

3 cups chopped tomatoes

½ cup chopped green bell pepper

1 cup onion, diced

¼ cup minced fresh cilantro

2 tablespoons fresh lime juice

4 teaspoons chopped fresh jalapeno pepper (including seeds)

½ teaspoon ground cumin

½ teaspoon kosher salt

½ teaspoon ground black pepper

Directions

Step 1

Stir the tomatoes, green bell pepper, onion, cilantro, lime juice, jalapeno pepper, cumin, salt, and pepper in a bowl. Serve.

Nutrition Facts

Per Serving: 5 calories; protein 0.2g; carbohydrates 1.1g; sodium 25.1mg.

Easy Never Forgotten Guacamole

This guacamole has been a hit at our house for years. Great for the Superbowl or any occasion. Sour cream and cream cheese make the guac extra creamy. Spice it up with crushed red pepper.

Prep: 10 mins

Additional: 30 mins

Total: 40 mins

Servings: 16

Yield: 2 cups

Ingredients

3 avocados - peeled, pitted and diced

1 tablespoon sour cream

2 (3 ounce) packages cream cheese, softened

2 tablespoons salsa

1 pinch salt

1 dash ground black pepper

1 dash garlic salt

1 dash onion powder

Directions

Step 1

In a small bowl, mix together the avocados, sour cream, cream cheese and salsa. Blend to desired consistency.

Step 2

In a small bowl mix the salt, pepper, garlic salt and onion powder. Stir into the avocado mixture. Cover and chill in the refrigerator 1/2 hour before serving.

Nutrition Facts

Per Serving: 100 calories; protein 1.6g; carbohydrates 3.8g; fat 9.4g; cholesterol 12.1mg; sodium 67.4mg.

Amazing Chickpea Cinnamon Pancakes

Gluten-free, sugar-free, low-cholesterol, light and fluffy low-fat pancakes that taste great! Perfect for South Beach Diet® Phase One.

Prep: 15 mins

Cook: 5 mins

Total: 20 mins

Servings: 6

Yield: 8 pancakes

Ingredients

1 cup chickpea (garbanzo bean) flour

1 tablespoon ground cinnamon

2 teaspoons baking powder

4 (1 gram) packets stevia powder

¼ teaspoon salt

1 cup nonfat milk

¼ cup beaten egg whites

2 tablespoons vegetable oil

Directions

Step 1

Mix chickpea flour, cinnamon, baking powder, stevia powder, and salt together in a bowl.

Step 2

Whisk milk, egg whites, and vegetable oil together in a separate bowl. Pour over the chickpea flour mixture; whisk until batter is just combined.

Step 3

Heat a lightly oiled griddle over medium-high heat. Pour 1/2 cup portions onto the griddle and cook until bubbles form and the edges are dry, 3 to 4 minutes. Flip and cook until browned on the other side, 2 to 3 minutes. Repeat with remaining batter.

Nutrition Facts

Per Serving: 180 calories; protein 8.4g; carbohydrates 19.8g; fat 8.4g; cholesterol 1.2mg; sodium 440.3mg.

Crispy Jacket Potatoes

These crispy jacket potatoes are like a baked potato, but better. Serve with butter and sour cream.

Crispy jacket potatoes topped with sour cream and chives on a platter.

Prep Time: 10 mins

Cook Time: 1 hr

Total Time: 1 hr 10 mins

Servings: 6

Yield: 6 potatoes

Ingredients

6 medium russet potatoes

1 tablespoon vegetable oil, or as needed

¼ teaspoon sea salt, or to taste

1 pinch lemon-pepper seasoning, or to taste

12 large squares aluminum foil

Directions

Gather ingredients. Preheat the oven to 400 degrees F (200 degrees C).

Various ingredients for crispy jacket potatoes.

Drizzle potatoes with a thin layer of oil. Sprinkle on sea salt and about 1/2 as much lemon-pepper seasoning.

Whole potatoes seasoned with salt and pepper.

Wrap each potato in a square of foil, then wrap with a second square. Place foil-wrapped potatoes in a glass or ceramic baking dish.

Foil wrapped potatoes in a casserole dish.

Bake in the preheated oven until the skins are crisp and the flesh is soft, 60 to 90 minutes.

Baked potatoes on a white plate.

Serve with butter, sour cream, or any of your favorite toppings!

Crispy jacket potatoes topped with sour cream and chives on a platter.

Conclusion

In addition to incorporating plenty of heart-healthy foods into your diet, it's important to take a look at the rest of your diet as well. The majority of your diet should consist of unprocessed, whole foods, such as fruits, vegetables, meats and whole grains.

When you're grocery shopping, stick to the outer sections of the store, and avoid wandering into the middle where the heavily processed junk foods lurk.

Be sure to also opt for healthy fats when you're cooking or baking. Skip the vegetable oils, margarine and shortening, and choose nutrient-rich coconut oil, extra-virgin olive oil, butter or ghee instead.

For those with high blood pressure, limiting your sodium intake is also critical. Steer clear of fast food, frozen meals and convenience foods, all of which can be hidden sources of sodium.

If this all seems overwhelming, no worries. Start by making one small change each week, and you'll work your way up to a healthy, well-rounded diet in no time!

Although these foods may be associated with some impressive health benefits, chowing down on a few walnuts per day won't make much of a difference if the rest of your diet is filled with ultra-processed foods.

Use these heart-healthy foods to round out a nutritious diet filled with fruits, vegetables, proteins, whole grains and healthy fats. Additionally, make sure to combine them with an active lifestyle, minimal stress levels and adequate sleep.

If you do have heart problems, be sure to talk to your doctor and pair these heart-healthy foods with your treatment plan to maximize your results and see the most benefit to your health.